# In the Hands of Eternity

ALVIN T. HARMON II

# DEDICATION

To all who struggle with the promises God has made concerning the end of human life. I pray you find the peace necessary to return the vessel you were given.

In the Hands of Eternity

# TABLE OF CONTENTS

# Part 1: Destined to Die

---

## *Introduction: Facing the Inevitable*

"To every reader of this book, I have some news that may be alarming: we die. I don't mean to shock you, but I want us to begin with this undeniable truth. Each one of us, without exception, will face the moment when we separate from this physical world."

We often live as if life will continue indefinitely. We plan, we worry, and we strive, often without pausing to consider that one day, our names will also be inscribed on a gravestone. I remember, long before my work in end-of-life care, a day that profoundly shifted my view on life and mortality. I was just a propane delivery driver at the time, making a stop at an old church in the woods. That day, as I stood by the stained glass of that humble chapel, I looked out over a modest but crowded graveyard, where row upon row of stones marked lives that had passed.

Looking at the names on those stones, I wondered what faces went with those names. Who were they? What dreams and fears did they have? What conversations did they share, and who remembered them now? I was suddenly struck by the revelation that one day—maybe soon, maybe far off—my own name would be carved into a stone much like those, another life remembered by others. It was a thought that shook me to my core but also brought me peace. I realized then that my time here was part of a much greater cycle—one that no person has ever avoided, from the humblest to the most powerful.

The Bible brings this point home beautifully in Hebrews 9:27–28: *"Just as people are destined to die once, and after that to face judgment, so Christ was sacrificed once to take away the sins of many; and He will appear a second time, not to bear sin, but to bring salvation to those who are waiting for Him."*

The notion of destiny often brings to mind something beautiful or exciting, yet we hesitate to see death as part of that destiny. But what if we viewed it differently? Instead of dreading it, we could embrace it as part of a journey that leads to the peace of salvation promised in Christ.

---

### *Reflection: Understanding the Value of Mortality*

As we begin this journey together, I invite you to reflect on what your own life might look like when seen through the lens of mortality. How does the reality that one day your name will be remembered in this way change the way you live now? So often, it's only when we come face to face with our limited time that we gain clarity about what truly matters.

Here's an exercise: take a few quiet moments and think about the most meaningful memories in your life. What have you loved, created, or contributed that you'd like to be remembered by? Perhaps even write down a few reflections or memories. Let this be a grounding reminder as we continue through the pages ahead.

### *Embracing Mortality as Part of God's Plan*

It may be tempting to avoid these thoughts or even reject them as too uncomfortable, but acknowledging our mortality brings perspective. And this isn't just an individual journey; it's one that all of humanity shares. We are connected by our common destiny of life, death, and eternity. By understanding this, we gain not only peace but also the ability to truly live.

*"For everything there is a season, and a time for every matter under heaven: a time to be born, and a time to die..."* (Ecclesiastes 3:1–2). Here we see that every season of life has its place in God's perfect order. Death, too, has a place—a completion that brings our physical story to an end but opens the door to eternity. With this perspective, we can begin to view our journey toward the end of life not with fear, but with acceptance, knowing it's been "destined" for each of us by God Himself.

Death is not a thief, taking away what is ours; it's a bridge leading us into the fullness of our eternal purpose. Our journey will continue on the other side of this life in ways we cannot yet understand.

### *A Prayer for Embracing Our Mortality*

I invite you now to join in a brief prayer, inviting God's presence and peace to fill your heart as you reflect on the cycle of life He has set in place.

*"Father, we thank You for the gift of life. We recognize that we are only here for a time, and that time is precious. Help us to accept this reality not with fear, but with gratitude and peace. Guide our hearts and minds as we reflect on the meaning and purpose You have given each of us. Help us embrace every season of life, knowing that Your promise of eternity awaits us. Amen."*

### *Chapter Takeaway*

As we conclude this chapter, let's carry forward a simple truth: **death is not a tragic end, but a part of a journey that leads us to our eternal home**. When we embrace this, we open ourselves to live with intention, meaning, and a greater appreciation for each moment.

# Part 2: What It Means to Die

---

## *Introduction: Beyond the Physical Body*

In the Western world, death is often defined only as a physical end—a moment when the body stops functioning. But within a biblical framework, death is much more than that. It is a separation, yes, but it is also a reunion and a transformation. It's the journey where the spirit, soul, and body part ways, as the body returns to the earth, the soul finds rest, and the spirit returns to God.

*"Then shall the dust return to the earth as it was: and the spirit shall return unto God who gave it."* (Ecclesiastes 12:7, KJV)

Here, we find a truth that has been present in scripture for millennia: death is simply the separation of these parts that make up the whole of who we are. This separation allows our spiritual essence—our eternal self—to return to its Creator, while the body, which has been our vessel on Earth, returns to the dust. In a way, death is a homecoming for the soul, a chance to reunite with the One who formed it.

### *Understanding the Three Parts: Spirit, Soul, and Body*

The Bible speaks of each person as having three essential parts: the body, the soul, and the spirit. These three are closely knit together, working in harmony throughout our lives, but in death, they go their separate ways.

1. **The Body**: Our bodies are the physical structures that allow us to move, breathe, and interact with the world. They carry the memories of our experiences, hold the marks of our work, and show the effects of time. But the body is only temporary—a vessel for our time on earth.
2. **The Soul**: The soul can be understood as the seat of our emotions, thoughts, and will. It's the part of us that feels, desires, and remembers. Our soul holds our unique personality, shaped by our choices and experiences.
3. **The Spirit**: The spirit is the divine spark within us—the part that connects directly to God. When we die, it is this spirit that returns to its Source, reuniting with the One who breathed life into us at the beginning.

In 1 Thessalonians 5:23, Paul prays for the sanctification of these three aspects: *"May your whole spirit, soul, and body be kept blameless at the coming of our Lord Jesus Christ."* This distinction between spirit, soul, and body reminds us that while our bodies may rest in the earth, our spirit and soul continue beyond the grave.

---

### A Peaceful Separation

When death comes, it is not a violent ripping away but a peaceful release. Just as a loved one falls asleep, the spirit leaves the body, and the soul finds peace. David speaks to this in Psalm 116:15: *"Precious in the sight of the Lord is the death of His saints."* There is nothing to fear in this separation because, in God's eyes, death is a moment of precious transition, a homecoming.

As believers, this separation should bring comfort rather than fear. To think of death as a peaceful release, a returning of the spirit to God, allows us to face the idea of death without dread. It is merely the end of our earthly journey and the beginning of our eternity.

### The Beauty of Eternal Transition

In death, we do not lose who we are; rather, we become fully who God has intended us to be in Him. The Apostle Paul writes in 2 Corinthians 5:8, *"We are confident, I say, and would prefer to be away from the body and at home with the Lord."* He understood that being with the Lord was the ultimate destination for our spirit and soul.

Death, then, is not just an end; it's a fulfillment of the life of faith we've been called to. We move from the temporary to the eternal, from the limited to the boundless presence of God.

Here's a reflection exercise: consider a moment in your life when you felt truly at peace. Imagine that peace expanded infinitely and without end. This is only a glimpse of the peace we are promised when our spirit is with God.

### *Facing the Journey Together*

Scripture tells us that we are never alone, even in death. Psalm 23:4 offers this reassurance: *"Even though I walk through the valley of the shadow of death, I will fear no evil, for You are with me; Your rod and Your staff, they comfort me."* God promises to be with us through every step, guiding our spirit homeward.

For those left behind, knowing that our loved one's spirit has been welcomed by God is a profound comfort. Death, though painful, becomes an act of entrusting our loved one into the arms of a faithful and loving Creator.

### *Prayer for Peace in Separation*

Let's take a moment to pray for peace as we meditate on this mystery of death—the separation of the spirit, soul, and body:

*"Heavenly Father, we thank You for the spirit within us that You so lovingly created. We acknowledge that in Your divine wisdom, our spirit, soul, and body serve their purpose for a time and that one day they will part ways as we transition to eternity. May we find peace in this truth, knowing that our spirit will be safely in Your care. Help us, Lord, to release our fears and anxieties about death and to trust in Your perfect plan for us. Amen."*

### *Chapter Takeaway*

As we complete this chapter, let's carry forward this insight: **death is not an end to who we are but a continuation of who we are in Christ**. Our spirit returns to its Creator, and we experience the ultimate peace in His presence.

# Part 3: Betta' Not Talk About It

## Introduction: The Unspoken Topic

In many African American Christian households, death is a topic wrapped in silence. We may fear talking about it, as if speaking its name might invite it closer. For some, even bringing it up feels like bad luck, while for others, it's a topic reserved only for funerals and moments of grief. Yet, avoiding it does not make it disappear; it only makes us less prepared.

Imagine the peace that might come if, instead of avoiding the conversation, we embraced it with faith. We can discover a sense of preparedness, grounded in our belief that God's promise extends beyond this life. By opening the conversation, we allow ourselves to understand death in a healthier, faith-centered way, seeing it not as an end but as a transition in God's plan.

## Facing the Fear of Death

In the African American community, our cultural history has often led us to adopt a sense of quiet resilience. Yet, the pain and trauma of that history have also shaped a protective silence around death. When life has been fragile, when people have endured oppression and loss, discussing death can feel like inviting additional hardship. But avoiding the subject doesn't change its reality; it only leaves us unprepared for its inevitability.

For many, death has become the "enemy" of life—a perspective that blocks us from seeing it as a natural and necessary part of our journey. It is essential to remember that even Christ himself embraced death as a step toward resurrection and victory. *"Even though I walk through the valley of the shadow of death, I will fear no evil, for You are with me."* (Psalm 23:4)

This verse reassures us that we don't need to walk in fear. Rather, we can face the topic with strength, comforted by the knowledge that God walks with us, even in our final journey.

---

### *The Cultural Silence on Death*

Silence around death in the African American Christian faith community often stems from historical and emotional roots. Generations past may not have had the resources to plan or discuss end-of-life arrangements, and conversations about death could feel like they were courting disaster. These barriers have grown into an unspoken rule: "betta' not talk about it." By challenging this silence, we free ourselves to view death through the lens of faith rather than fear.

In many churches, we speak of resurrection and eternal life, but we don't often dwell on the actual process of dying. We avoid talking about the physical end as if it's a contradiction to God's plan for us. Yet scripture reminds us that life and death are both integral parts of God's design. Paul tells us in *Philippians 1:21,* "For to me, to live is Christ and to die is gain." He didn't fear death; he saw it as a gain—a step closer to being with God.

---

### *Breaking the Silence Together*

As a community, we can reclaim this conversation. Imagine a future where our families and congregations speak openly about life's end without fear. Breaking the silence allows us to approach this part of life with dignity and faith.

Here are ways to begin shifting this perspective:

1. **Start with the Church**: Faith leaders can play a powerful role in setting a tone that normalizes conversations about death. Sermons that address death openly from a biblical perspective can help open doors for healthy discussions within congregations.
2. **Talk Within Families**: Sharing thoughts about death with family members builds trust and connection. By discussing personal beliefs, preferences, and questions, families

can grow closer and find comfort in mutual understanding.

3. **Create Supportive Spaces**: Community groups, prayer circles, or even informal gatherings can become safe spaces to share feelings about death. These meetings can foster compassion and understanding, helping people feel supported through the journey.

---

### Finding Peace in Faith

When we bring death into the light of our faith, it loses its power to scare us. We begin to understand it not as a destructive force but as a transformative one, leading us closer to God's presence. John 11:25, *"I am the resurrection and the life. The one who believes in me will live, even though they die,"* reminds us that, for believers, death is not a final defeat but the beginning of a new, eternal chapter.

---

### Closing Prayer

*"Heavenly Father, You who are the beginning and the end, we thank You for the gift of life and the promise of eternal peace. Give us the courage to speak of death with open hearts, free from fear. Help us to embrace this journey as part of Your divine plan, knowing that You are with us in life and*

*in death. Let our faith guide us and let our love for one another give us strength. Amen."*

---

### Chapter Summary

Talking about death doesn't take away from life—it adds meaning to it. By breaking the silence, we begin to see death not as a threat but as a transition to God's promised peace.

# Part 4: The Struggle

---

### Introduction: A Difficult Truth to Embrace

As we journey through life, it's natural to celebrate beginnings—births, new relationships, fresh starts. But scripture offers us a surprising perspective on the end of life. Ecclesiastes 7:1 tells us, *"A good name is better than fine perfume, and the day of death better than the day of birth."* This verse presents a challenge to our usual view of life and death, especially for those of us in faith communities that traditionally revere life's beginnings and often avoid facing its end.

It's understandable; to the human mind, death can seem like loss, the end of a cherished story. But this verse offers a glimpse into how God's view may differ from ours. In God's eyes, a well-lived life fulfilled in death can be even more precious than its beginning. This chapter will explore what it means to embrace this challenging truth and how we can learn to see the day of our passing as a fulfillment rather than a defeat.

## Life's Cycle: The Three Parts of a Pencil

Imagine life as a pencil. When we look at it, we see three main parts: the eraser, the wood, and the graphite core. Each has its purpose, and none exists without the others. Our existence is much like this pencil: birth is like the fresh, sharpened point, our years of living are the wood that holds us together, and death is the eraser that completes the pencil's purpose.

As strange as it might sound, the eraser is just as important as the wood and the graphite; it's what allows the pencil to fulfill its purpose and start again anew. In this way, death is not an opponent to life—it's a part of the process that brings meaning and completion.

From this perspective, Ecclesiastes 7:1 encourages us to value the "day of death" because it completes life's purpose. Through our faith, we begin to see that death isn't the end; it's the last chapter in a story well-lived, a chapter that leads us closer to God.

## Understanding "Better than Birth"

Why does Ecclesiastes say that the day of death is "better than the day of birth"? At birth, our life is a blank slate, a promise waiting to unfold. By the time of our passing, we have lived, loved, struggled, and learned. We've grown, developed character, and perhaps even left a legacy. Death, then, is the culmination of a lifetime of experiences.

In faith, we can see death as a reward for a life faithfully lived. The Bible promises us peace and rest after a journey that has tested and grown us. Our death is not a retreat from life but an entry into the eternal presence of God.

## Embracing the Beauty of Life's Completion

For those of us in faith communities, this perspective can feel challenging. Death often brings sorrow, separation, and grief. However, when we look beyond the immediate loss, we find something profound: the beauty of life's completion. Psalm 116:15 states, *"Precious in the sight of the Lord is the death of His faithful servants."* For God, our death is not a loss but a gain—a homecoming.

This passage reminds us that our death is precious to God because it represents our return to Him, our fulfillment of His plan. We live our lives on earth as His servants, and death is the moment we are called home. It is not an enemy but a reunion, a moment of joy in God's sight.

---

### A New Understanding of Legacy

Ecclesiastes 7:1 also reminds us that *"a good name is better than fine perfume."* Throughout our lives, we build our character, and that character—our reputation, our integrity, our kindness—becomes our legacy. Just as a fine fragrance lingers in a room, a good name leaves a lasting impact on the world, one that doesn't fade with our passing.

When we live with integrity, love, and faith, we leave behind something of value, something that brings meaning to the day of our death. In this way, death is a continuation of life's impact, a mark we leave that lives on in others.

### *Living in Peace with Death*

Accepting death as part of life's cycle helps us to live with peace. It shifts our focus from fearing the end to making the most of the present. When we stop viewing death as the ultimate defeat, we become free to see it as a step in a much larger journey.

By embracing this biblical wisdom, we can learn to live with a spirit of peace, valuing each day and trusting that God will be with us in the final chapter, guiding us into His eternal presence. Ecclesiastes 3:1-2 reminds us, *"There is a time for everything, and a season for every activity under the heavens: a time to be born and a time to die."*

If we can accept that there is a time for everything, we can begin to see death as God's appointed time for us—a time not to resist but to embrace as part of His plan.

---

### *Closing Prayer*

*"Lord, You are the giver of life, and You alone determine our time here on earth. Help us to live with faith, to embrace each day, and to trust in Your plan. May we find comfort in knowing that our lives have meaning in You, and that when our journey ends, we will find peace in Your presence. Grant us*

*the wisdom to see death not as an end but as a homecoming. Amen."*

---

### Chapter Summary

Death may challenge our human understanding, but in faith, we can see it as part of life's beautiful design. It is the moment when our story reaches its full meaning, and our legacy continues to inspire others.

## Part 5: Believe in a Better Day

---

### Introduction: Finding Peace in the Promise

The thought of leaving this world can often bring fear and sorrow, even for people of faith. But what if we could see beyond the veil of death to the promise waiting on the other side? What if, rather than fearing the end, we embraced it as a doorway to a better day—a day filled with peace, reunion, and joy in God's presence? Scripture reminds us that we have not been left without hope. As we explore these promises, let's open our hearts to what it truly means to believe in a better day.

### Death as a Passage, Not an End

In John 14:1-3, Jesus offers comfort by saying, *"Do not let your hearts be troubled. You believe in God; believe also in Me. My Father's house has many rooms... I am going there to prepare a place for you."* These words reflect a profound truth: death is not an end but a passage. Jesus assures us that we are simply moving from one room to another, from this temporary world to an eternal home prepared just for us.

By framing death as a transition, Jesus shifts our perspective from fear to anticipation. When we face life's end, we are not closing a door but stepping through one. This promise can change our entire outlook, allowing us to face death with peace, knowing we are moving toward something better.

### The Gift of Eternal Life

One of the most powerful promises of faith is the gift of eternal life. John 3:16 declares, *"For God so loved the world that He gave His one and only Son,*

*that whoever believes in Him shall not perish but
have eternal life."* This verse is more than a
comfort; it's a promise that life doesn't end with our
last breath. Rather, it continues in a new,
unimaginable form, free from pain, suffering, and
sorrow.

Eternal life isn't merely an extension of our earthly
existence—it's a transformation into a life filled
with the fullness of God's love and presence. With
this assurance, we find courage to live fully today,
knowing that tomorrow holds something even
greater.

### The Peace That Passes Understanding

Philippians 4:7 speaks of the "peace of God, which
transcends all understanding." This peace is one of
the great promises of faith, especially when facing
death. It's not a peace that comes from our
circumstances or even our strength; it's a divine
peace that comes only from God. This peace
enables us to look at life's most challenging
moments, even death, and know that all will be
well.

When we surrender our fears to God, we open
ourselves to this peace. We stop clinging to life as if
it's all we have, trusting instead that God has
something better in store. With this peace, death no

longer feels like a loss but a passage into a peace that is beyond our comprehension.

---

### A Vision of Heaven

Revelation 21:4 gives us a vision of heaven, describing it as a place where *"He will wipe every tear from their eyes. There will be no more death or mourning or crying or pain, for the old order of things has passed away."* These words offer a glimpse into the life waiting beyond this world—a life untouched by sorrow, fear, or pain.

This promise reminds us that heaven is not just a place; it's a state of perfect peace and joy in God's presence. In heaven, our souls are restored, and our hearts find complete fulfillment in Him. With this image of heaven, we can face death with confidence, knowing that we are moving toward a place of perfect love and peace.

### Hope for Those Left Behind

While faith provides comfort to those facing death, it also offers hope to those left behind. First Thessalonians 4:13-14 encourages believers to grieve, but not without hope, saying, *"Brothers and sisters, we do not want you to be uninformed about those who sleep in death, so that you do not grieve like the rest of mankind, who have no hope."*

This passage acknowledges the pain of loss but assures us that it is not without hope. In the Christian faith, death is a temporary separation, a waiting period until we are reunited in God's eternal presence. This promise of reunion can be a source of strength for those mourning, reminding them that love transcends even death.

---

### *Living with Expectation*

As we live our lives, we can hold onto the expectation that there is something beautiful and meaningful waiting for us. This perspective transforms how we live today. When we know that a better day is coming, we can live with purpose, make peace with our fears, and focus on what truly matters.

The Apostle Paul captures this spirit of expectation in 2 Timothy 4:7-8, saying, *"I have fought the good fight, I have finished the race, I have kept the faith. Now there is in store for me the crown of righteousness, which the Lord, the righteous Judge, will award to me on that day."* Paul's words reflect a life lived in expectation of the ultimate reward, a "better day" that makes every struggle, sacrifice, and challenge worthwhile.

### *Letting Go of Fear, Embracing Faith*

In this journey, letting go of fear becomes an act of faith. Rather than clinging to life, we place our trust in God's promises. We may not know exactly what lies beyond, but we know the One who awaits us there. As Jesus said in John 11:25, *"I am the resurrection and the life. The one who believes in Me will live, even though they die."*

This verse isn't just a promise; it's an invitation to trust. Jesus invites us to believe not only in Him but also in the life He offers, one that surpasses even death. When we release our fear of the unknown, we find ourselves free to live and love with an open heart, trusting that God's promises hold true.

### *Living in Light of a Better Day*

As we reflect on these promises, we are called to live each day in the light of eternity. This doesn't mean ignoring life's difficulties or bypassing grief; it means trusting that even in our most challenging moments, there is something greater waiting. The better day that God promises is not just a distant hope; it's a reality that shapes our lives here and now, giving us purpose, peace, and joy.

By living in light of this promise, we honor God's gift of life and prepare ourselves for the eternal joy that awaits. We can walk through life's valleys without fear, knowing that the best is yet to come.

### Closing Prayer

*"Heavenly Father, we thank You for the promises of peace and hope that You have given us. Help us to live each day with the knowledge that death is not the end but the beginning of something beautiful. May we trust in Your love, surrender our fears, and walk in the light of Your promises. Give us courage and faith as we face life's uncertainties, knowing that a better day is coming. Amen."*

---

### Chapter Summary

This chapter reminds us that death is not an end, but a promise fulfilled—a gateway to a day without sorrow, where God's peace is complete. By embracing this promise, we find the courage to live fully and love deeply, grounded in the certainty of a better day that lies ahead.

## Part 6: Beyond Goodbye

*Introduction: A Life That Speaks Beyond Words*

In every life, there is a story unfolding—a narrative shaped by our choices, words, and actions. These stories often resonate beyond our presence, continuing to touch those we leave behind. This chapter reflects on what it means to create a legacy, not just in what we accumulate or accomplish, but in the kindness, we show, the love we give, and the wisdom we pass on. We all leave something behind, and how we live today can shape what that "something" will be for those who follow.

*Understanding Legacy: What We Leave Behind*

Legacy isn't about material wealth or public achievements alone. In Proverbs 13:22, we read, *"A good person leaves an inheritance for their children's children."* This verse speaks not only of physical inheritance but also of the values, love, and wisdom that we pass along. Our legacy is the culmination of how we've lived and loved, the lessons we've shared, and the lives we've touched. It's our opportunity to speak into the future, shaping the world in ways that reflect God's love and grace.

Consider the legacy of a loving parent, a compassionate friend, or a faithful servant. Each leaves behind a kind of spiritual inheritance that money can't buy—a legacy of faith, love, and wisdom that blesses those who remember them. When we choose to live intentionally, we create a legacy that reflects God's heart, shaping the lives of those who follow.

### Living with Purpose Today

To leave a legacy of impact, we must live with purpose now. Psalm 90:12 encourages us, *"Teach us to number our days, that we may gain a heart of wisdom."* This scripture isn't about fearing the end; it's about recognizing the value of each day and living it to the fullest. Each choice, each interaction, and each moment has meaning when we live intentionally.

Living with purpose means approaching life with a sense of mission. It's about seeking ways to serve, love, and encourage others. It's about using our talents, time, and resources to bring light and hope. By doing so, we leave behind something more valuable than possessions—a legacy of faith and goodness that points others toward God.

### *Words That Last: Speaking Life*

The words we speak hold power, echoing long after we've left. Proverbs 18:21 reminds us, *"The tongue has the power of life and death."* The words we choose today can either lift people up or tear them down; they can bring comfort, encouragement, and guidance. A kind word can inspire someone for a lifetime, and a word of wisdom can shape someone's future.

When we speak life into others, we leave a legacy of love and encouragement. We build them up, remind them of their worth, and point them toward God's love. Each word we speak has the potential to become part of our legacy, echoing through the lives of those who carry our words in their hearts.

---

### *Living Beyond Yourself*

In John 15:12-13, Jesus says, *"My command is this: Love each other as I have loved you. Greater love has no one than this: to lay down one's life for one's friends."* Jesus teaches us that a life well-lived is one marked by selflessness. When we live beyond ourselves, we create a legacy of compassion, kindness, and grace.

Living beyond ourselves means embracing a heart of service, choosing to put others before ourselves, and extending God's love to everyone we meet.

This is the legacy of Christ—a legacy of selfless love that transformed the world. When we choose to live with this same selflessness, our lives continue to make an impact, shaping a world that reflects God's love long after we're gone.

---

## Memories That Shape the Heart

Our legacy is also built on the memories we create with those around us. Simple moments of laughter, listening, and love can become lasting memories that comfort and inspire others. Ecclesiastes 3:1 reminds us, *"There is a time for everything, and a season for every activity under the heavens."* Each season of life offers opportunities to create meaningful memories, moments that touch the hearts of those we love.

These memories often become treasures, reminders of love that offer comfort and inspiration long after we're gone. Whether it's a family tradition, a shared meal, or a simple conversation, these moments become part of our legacy, carrying our love and values into the future.

## A Legacy of Faith

As people of faith, one of the greatest gifts we can leave is a legacy of belief and trust in God. Second Timothy 4:7-8 expresses this beautifully: *"I have fought the good fight, I have finished the race, I have kept the faith. Now there is in store for me the crown of righteousness."* This passage reflects the heart of someone who has lived faithfully, passing along a legacy of belief that inspires future generations.

A legacy of faith is not about perfection but about commitment. It's the steady journey of trusting God through life's highs and lows, showing others the value of a life centered on Christ. When we share our faith through our words, actions, and prayers, we plant seeds of faith that can continue to grow long after we're gone.

---

### Carrying Love Forward

In First Corinthians 13:13, we are reminded that *"the greatest of these is love."* Love is the ultimate legacy. When we choose to love, we create something that lasts beyond our lifetime. Love is the one gift that remains, echoing in the hearts of those we leave behind.

A legacy of love is the most enduring inheritance we can offer. It's found in the kindness we show, the forgiveness we extend, and the grace we offer. When we love well, we leave behind a piece of ourselves that continues to bless others. Our love becomes a reminder of God's love, a light that shines even in our absence.

### *The Invitation to Build a Lasting Legacy*

Legacy isn't something we build overnight; it's something we create one day at a time. By choosing to live with purpose, to speak life, to serve others, and to love deeply, we create a legacy that reflects God's heart. We leave behind a story that inspires others to live fully, love deeply, and trust God's promises.

Today, we are invited to begin building this legacy. We can start by reaching out in kindness, speaking words of encouragement, and living with an open heart. Each choice we make becomes a chapter in our story, a part of the legacy we leave behind.

---

### *Closing Prayer*

*"Lord, help us to live each day with purpose, building a legacy that reflects Your love and grace. May our words and actions bring life and hope to those around us. Teach us to serve, to love, and to live with open hearts, knowing that the impact of our lives will echo in the hearts of those we leave behind. Help us to trust in Your promises and to believe that our legacy, grounded in faith, will point others to You. Amen."*

*Chapter Summary*

This chapter has been a reflection on the power of legacy. Our lives are like stained glass windows, shining in ways that bless and inspire others long after we're gone. By living with intention, loving deeply, and sharing our faith, we create a legacy that endures—a legacy that speaks of God's love and hope.

# Part 7: Eternal Perspectives

*Introduction: Faith for Every Moment, Faith for Eternity*

As we draw near to the end of this journey, we reflect on the continuous thread of faith that weaves through our lives. Life and death are deeply connected, not as adversaries but as parts of a single, divinely woven tapestry. The same faith that brings us hope, strength, and purpose in life is the faith that carries us with peace into eternity. This faith reassures us that life does not end with death but transforms into something greater—an everlasting life in the presence of God. Just as faith sustains us through every trial, it also prepares us for the final, eternal transition.

---

### Living with an Eternal Perspective

The Bible calls us to live with our eyes set on eternity, embracing this world while anticipating the next. Colossians 3:2 says, *"Set your minds on things above, not on earthly things."* Living with an eternal perspective means that we view life's experiences in light of God's ultimate plan. We recognize that every joy, sorrow, challenge, and triumph here is part of a larger, eternal story.

When we live with eternity in mind, we gain freedom from life's temporary concerns. Our faith becomes not just a source of strength for today but a preparation for the life to come. As we walk with God through life, we are assured that He will also walk with us through the doorway into eternity. Faith teaches us that, just as God has been faithful to sustain us in life, He is also faithful to carry us into His eternal presence.

### The Faith to Trust Beyond Time

Hebrews 11:1 tells us, *"Now faith is confidence in what we hope for and assurance about what we do not see."* Faith isn't limited to the things we can control or understand. It is the confidence to trust God beyond our time here, to place our lives—and our eternity—in His hands. We are reminded that our journey with God doesn't end with our final breath; it continues into eternity, where we will see Him face to face.

The faith it takes to live is the same faith it takes to die because both require a surrender of our fears and uncertainties into God's loving care. In life, faith allows us to navigate the unknowns, believing that God's hand is guiding us. In death, faith reassures us that God's hand will still be there, leading us into His eternal promises. Trusting God in life prepares us to trust Him in death, knowing that He who created us has also prepared a place for us.

---

### Embracing Peace through Faith

In John 14:27, Jesus offers a profound promise: *"Peace I leave with you; my peace I give you. I do not give to you as the world gives. Do not let your hearts be troubled and do not be afraid."* This peace is the assurance that God is with us, that He knows every step of our journey, and that His love covers both life and death. Faith in God's promises allow us to face life's end with the same peace and confidence we've sought throughout our days.

Peace comes when we trust that God's love and care are unfailing. We can let go of the anxieties and uncertainties that often surround death because we are held by the same God who has faithfully carried us through every season of life. This peace allows us to rest in the truth that death is not an end but a doorway into God's eternal presence.

---

### A Faith That Transcends Boundaries

One of the greatest gifts of faith is that it removes the boundaries between life and eternity. Second Corinthians 5:8 reminds us, *"We are confident, I say, and would prefer to be away from the body and at home with the Lord."* For those who trust in Christ, the journey doesn't end in death but continues in the presence of the One who loves us beyond measure.

Faith allows us to see beyond the visible, to trust that God's promises are true, even if they extend beyond our earthly understanding. This faith isn't a wishful hope; it's a certainty anchored in God's Word and His faithfulness. Death becomes not a wall, but a passageway into the fulfillment of His promises, where our faith meets sight, and we experience the fullness of God's love and glory.

### Living with Hope, Dying with Assurance

The Apostle Paul speaks to this assurance in Second Timothy 4:7-8: *"I have fought the good fight, I have finished the race, I have kept the faith. Now there is in store for me the crown of righteousness, which the Lord, the righteous Judge, will award to me on that day."* Paul's words remind us that a life lived with faith prepares us to face the end with assurance, knowing that we are stepping into God's eternal embrace.

When we embrace faith in both life and death, we are free to live each day with purpose and confidence. Our lives become a testament to God's faithfulness, and our transition into eternity becomes a final act of trust. In dying with faith, we enter into the promises God has prepared, confident that His love and grace will guide us home.

---

### Faith: The Bridge Between Earth and Heaven

Faith is the bridge that carries us from the temporal into the eternal. Psalm 23:4 beautifully illustrates this journey: *"Even though I walk through the valley of the shadow of death, I will fear no evil, for you are with me; your rod and your staff, they comfort me."* This scripture reassures us that God is with us, not only through the joys of life but also through the journey of passing into eternity. Faith is the steady presence of God that guides us, the trust that He will bring us safely into His kingdom.

As we cross the threshold of this life, we are reminded that faith is not only for the living; it's the foundation for our journey into God's eternal promises. The same faith that sustained us through life's trials and triumphs becomes our anchor as we move into eternity, knowing that God is with us in every step.

---

## A Final Prayer of Trust

*"Lord, we thank You for the gift of faith—a faith that guides us through life and prepares us for eternity. Help us to trust You in all things, knowing that Your love is constant, and Your promises are true. Give us peace in the face of life's end, confidence in Your promises, and joy in the assurance that we will be with You forever. Teach us to live each day with purpose and to face the unknown with a faith that rests in Your love. Amen."*

---

## Closing Thoughts on Faith and Eternity

This chapter has been an invitation to view life and death through the lens of faith, seeing both as parts of a continuous journey with God. We have been given the gift of faith, not only to sustain us through life but to guide us into eternity. The same faith that brings us courage in life becomes our peace in death, uniting us with God in love that transcends all boundaries.

---

In closing, may this journey through faith, life, and eternity inspire a deep and lasting trust in God's promises. As you turn the final pages, remember that life's journey is held in His hands, and our destination is secure in His eternal embrace. This faith, powerful enough to carry us through every challenge and joy, is the same faith that leads us home.

## Summary: A Journey of Faith, Life, and Eternity

*In the Hands of Eternity* has been a journey through some of life's most profound questions and mysteries. Together, we have explored the nature of faith, the beauty of life, and the peace that comes with embracing death not as an end but as a divine transition into God's eternal presence.

This book began with a look at the preciousness of life itself, likening it to stained glass—made from pieces that are individually beautiful, yet infinitely more compelling when seen together as a whole. Just as light shines through colored glass, our lives take on deeper meaning and purpose when we allow God's presence to illuminate us. This view invites us to see each experience, each joy, and each sorrow as a vital part of the greater masterpiece God is creating.

We journeyed through what it truly means to die, considering death not as the defeat of life but as its fulfillment. By understanding the separation of body, soul, and spirit, we're able to embrace death with hope rather than fear. We saw that death is the continuation of our relationship with God, one in which faith doesn't cease but instead carries us over the threshold of this life into His eternal presence.

Reflecting on the hesitancies and cultural taboos that sometimes hinder the African American Christian community from engaging in conversations about death, we examined the strength that comes from confronting these topics openly. These reflections guide us to see that death, like life, is part of a holistic walk with God—one that invites trust and courage every step of the way.

Through scripture, we explored perspectives on why the end of life, as Ecclesiastes reminds us, can be better than its beginning. We found meaning in the notion that life's purpose is completed in God's timing and that a day spent with Him in eternity is worth more than all our earthly experiences combined. This perspective reorients our fears and doubts, replacing them with faith-filled assurance that God's ultimate plan is one of love, grace, and eternal peace.

Finally, we arrived at the theme of enduring faith— the faith that sustains us in life and guides us into eternity. Just as the faith to live well is the same faith that prepares us to die well, we can rest in the confidence that God's hand is both our anchor in life and our gateway to eternity. As we transition from life into God's promised peace, we are invited to see this not as a loss, but as the culmination of a life fully surrendered to Him.

In the end, *In the Hands of Eternity* calls readers to live each moment with purpose, to see God's hand in all things, and to trust that the same God who has held us through life's journey will continue to hold us in eternity. May this book inspire you to embrace life with faith, meet death with peace, and live each day with the wisdom that only comes from knowing God.

www.ingramcontent.com/pod-product-compliance
Lightning Source LLC
Chambersburg PA
CBHW071937020426
42331CB00010B/2919